NEW GLUTEN FREE DIET FOR WOMEN

Enjoy Easy and Healthy Recipes with Your Family

Copyright © 2021 All rights reserved. No part of this publication may be reproduced, distributed, or transmitted in any formor by any means, including photocopying, recording, or other electronic or mechanical methods, without the prior written permission of the publisher, except in the case of brief quotations embodied in critical reviews and certain other noncommercial uses permitted by copyright law

Table of Contents

- INTRODUCTION
- An Overview of Celiac Disease
  - Symptoms of Celiac Disease
  - How Your Doctor Diagnoses Celiac Disease
  - How Celiac Disease Is Treated
- An Overview of the Gluten-Free Diet
  - Avoiding Accidental Gluten Exposure
  - How To Recover From Accidental Gluten Exposure
  - Surgeries and Specialist-Driven Procedures
  - Complementary Alternative Medicine (CAM
  - Coping With Celiac Disease
  - Coping With Emotions When You're Newly Gluten-Free
- An Overview of the Gluten-Free Diet
  - What Is Gluten
  - Why Eat Gluten-Free
  - What Foods Contain Gluten
- How to Start a Gluten-Free Diet
  - Avoid Trace Amounts
  - How to Go Gluten-Free
  - Gluten-Free Diet Benefits
- Makeup Brands That Offer Gluten-Free Options
  - Should I Buy Gluten-Free Makeup
  - Skin Conditions That Might Be a Sign of a Gluten Allergy
  - Gluten-Free Makeup Brands
- Top 9 Gluten-Free Grains
  - Gluten-Free Grains vs. Grains with Gluten
- How to Include Gluten-Free Grains in Your Diet + Gluten-Free Grain Recipes
  - Gluten-free grains recipes
  - Paleo Tortillas Recipe Corn-Free with Healthy Oils
  - Slow Cooker Chicken and Rice Recipe
  - Crockpot chicken and rice ingredients
  - Spinach Mushroom Quiche
  - Gluten-Free Impossibly Easy Breakfast Bake

- [Peanut Butter Banana Pancakes](#)
- [Zucchini-Ribbon "Lasagna"](#)
- [Cauliflower Pizza Crust](#)

INTRODUCTION

Gluten-free has evolved from a flashy diet trend into big business. To put this in perspective, market trends suggest that gluten-free could be worth as much as at 7.59 billion dollars by 2020. In some surveys, over 25% of people stated that they were looking to try to cut gluten out of their diet for health reasons.

The good news is that if you choose to live gluten-free, you have more options than ever. The other side of this coin is that when diets and trends hit the mainstream, it creates an atmosphere ripe for myths and misinterpretation. Read on to cut through the confusion and learn what a gluten-free diet entails and the concrete way that it can help you.

A Gluten-Free Diet is a diet completely free of gluten. Gluten is a protein found in most grains (specifically those that include rye, barley, or wheat). A Gluten-Free diet is required for sufferers of Celiac disease – a disease that affects the small intestine and interferes with absorption of nutrients from food. People can have different degrees of gluten sensitivity ranging from minor digestive issues, wheat allergies, and IBS to severe Celiac disease.

Glutenous grains have also been linked to obesity and diabetes, but this is likely due to the fact that processed white wheat flour is in an abundance of products and it's also usually combined with sugar. Proponents of Ancestral diets claim that the human body has never evolved to eat glutinous grains which is why wheat is linked to so many health problems including obesity.

If you're diagnosed with celiac disease or non-celiac gluten sensitivity, you'll need to learn how to eat gluten-free, since doing so is essential to your long-term health. Or, you may decide to try a gluten-free diet even without a diagnosis—you may believe gluten-free may help you lose weight or improve another health condition you have.

Regardless of your reasons for choosing a gluten-free diet, this can be a tricky diet with a massive learning curve, especially at first. But if you follow the instructions and guidelines in this book in order you should be well on your way to safely eating gluten-free.

An Overview of Celiac Disease

Celiac disease is an autoimmune disease in which eating foods that contain the protein gluten—found in wheat, barley, and rye—causes damage to your small intestine. It has a wide range of potential symptoms. People who have untreated celiac disease often cannot absorb nutrients from their food, and this can lead to serious health complications, such as malnutrition, osteoporosis, infertility, and even cancer. Fortunately, the damage caused by celiac disease often can be reversed once you've been diagnosed and begin following a gluten-free diet, which is the only current treatment for the condition.

In celiac disease, gluten ingestion triggers your white blood cells to attack the lining of your small intestine. The lining of your small intestine is made up of tiny, finger-like projections called villi. The autoimmune reaction in celiac disease attacks those little fingers, ultimately eroding the intestinal lining until it's worn smooth. Since your villi help you digest foods, losing them to celiac disease leads to major problems.

Symptoms of Celiac Disease

The best-known (but not necessarily most common) symptoms of celiac disease include smelly diarrhea, abdominal pain, weight loss, and fatigue. However, celiac disease can affect just about every system in your body, including your skin, your hormones, and your bones and joints. It can cause symptoms you might never think to associate with the condition.

It's doubtful that there's a truly typical case of celiac disease; the condition can affect too many body systems for any one set of symptoms to be considered typical. Women, men, babies, and children are likely to experience celiac disease in quite divergent ways. And sometimes, you might have full-blown celiac but not have any symptoms at all.

Frequent Symptoms

The symptoms will vary considerably from person to person and are also significantly different for children and for adults.

Adults

Adult digestive symptoms may include:

Diarrhea

Constipation

Heartburn

Bloating

Flatulence

Nausea and vomiting

Weight loss

Abdominal pain

Approximately half of adults have non-digestive symptoms, which may include:

Iron-deficiency anemia

Fatigue

Bone or joint pain, arthritis

Bone loss

Itchy skin rash with blisters (dermatitis herpetiformis)

Mouth ulcers

Headaches

Peripheral neuropathy with numbness or tingling in the feet and hands

Anxiety or depression

Irregular menstrual cycle, infertility

Children

Celiac disease usually has digestive symptoms in children and infants. The most common symptoms are:

Abdominal bloating and pain

Chronic diarrhea

Vomiting

Constipation

Stool that is pale, foul-smelling, or fatty (floating)

Weight loss

Fatigue

Mood changes, irritability

Damage to dental enamel of the permanent teeth

Slowed growth, short height, delayed puberty

failure to thrive

Attention deficit hyperactivity disorder (ADHD)

Here's a breakdown of celiac disease symptoms and related conditions, categorized by the body system they affect.

Digestive Symptoms

Not everyone who's diagnosed with celiac disease experiences digestive symptoms, but many do. Still, these digestive symptoms can be subtle, and you might not necessarily associate them with celiac disease.

Chronic diarrhea is one hallmark symptom of celiac disease, and it appears to affect half or more of those newly diagnosed.

Frequently, the diarrhea is watery, smelly, and voluminous, and floats rather than sinks. However, plenty of people with celiac disease tend to have constipation rather than diarrhea, and some see their symptoms alternate between the two.2

Digestive symptoms can include diarrhea, constipation, heartburn, bloating, flatulence, nausea and even vomiting in certain circumstances. People with celiac disease often are diagnosed with irritable bowel syndrome.

In addition, other types of digestive symptoms can appear. For example, flatulence and excessive gas are common, as is abdominal bloating (many people describe themselves as looking "six months pregnant"). It's also common to have abdominal pain, which can be severe at times.

Additional digestive symptoms of celiac disease can include heartburn and reflux (some people already have been told they have gastroesophageal reflux disease or GERD), nausea and vomiting, and lactose intolerance. Undiagnosed celiacs sometimes develop pancreatitis or gallbladder disease, and many already have been diagnosed with irritable bowel syndrome (those IBS symptoms often lessen or disappear completely following a celiac disease diagnosis).

In addition, not everyone loses weight as an undiagnosed celiac. In fact, many people find they gain weight prior to diagnosis. Some people report being absolutely unable to shed excess pounds, no matter how much they diet and exercise.

Neurological Symptoms

Many people with undiagnosed celiac experience extreme fatigue that prevents them from performing everyday tasks and impacts their quality of life. Generally, fatigue seems to creep up on you, making it easy to blame it on getting older (as opposed to a treatable medical condition).

At the same time, insomnia and other sleep disorders are very common in people with celiac. It's the worst of both worlds: You're exhausted during the day but can't fall asleep or stay asleep at night.

It's not uncommon for people with celiac disease to experience headaches (including migraines), brain fog, fatigue, and insomnia. They also may have pins and needles in their hands and feet, feelings of dizziness, and depression and anxiety.

In addition, many people with celiac disease get "brain fog" due to gluten. When you have brain fog, you have trouble thinking clearly—it literally feels as if your brain is operating in a fog. You might have

trouble coming up with the right words to carry on an intelligent conversation, or you might misplace your car keys or fumble other common household tasks.

Some newly diagnosed celiacs already have diagnoses of migraine headaches; in many cases (but not all), these headaches will lessen in severity and frequency or even clear up completely once you adopt a gluten-free diet.6

Psychological symptoms such as depression, anxiety, attention-deficit hyperactivity disorder, and irritability occur frequently in people with undiagnosed celiac disease. In fact, long-diagnosed celiacs often can tell they've been exposed to gluten through their irritability—that symptom can appear within hours of exposure and linger for several days. In small children with celiac disease, sometimes irritability is the only symptom.

Peripheral neuropathy, in which you experience numbness, a sensation of pins and needles, and potentially weakness in your extremities, is one of the most frequently reported neurological symptoms of celiac disease. In addition, some people are diagnosed with gluten ataxia, which is brain damage characterized by the loss of balance and coordination that's due to gluten consumption. Restless leg syndrome has been reported as a common symptom of celiac disease.

Skin Disorders

You might see signs of celiac disease in your largest organ: your skin. Up to one-fourth of people with celiac suffer from dermatitis herpetiformis (a.k.a. "the gluten rash"), an intensely itchy skin rash. If you have dermatitis herpetiformis plus positive celiac blood tests, you have celiac disease—no further testing required.

dermatitis herpetiformis on legs and feet

People with celiac disease also may have a variety of other skin problems, including psoriasis, eczema, alopecia areata (an autoimmune condition where you lose your hair), hives, and even such common problems as acne and dry skin. There's no firm evidence that gluten ingestion causes or contributes to these skin problems, but the gluten-free diet helps clear them up in some cases.

Bone and Joint Symptoms

Bone and joint issues such as osteoporosis, joint pain, bone pain, rheumatoid arthritis, and fibromyalgia also occur with regularity in those with celiac disease. It's not clear what the connection is; it may involve nutritional deficiencies related to the fact that celiac causes intestinal damage, which makes it difficult for you to absorb vitamins and minerals. In some cases, the gluten-free diet can alleviate pain from these conditions.

Dental Issues

People with celiac disease often have terrible teeth and problematic gums. In adults with undiagnosed celiac disease, frequent cavities, eroding enamel, and other recurring dental problems can signal the condition. Children with undiagnosed celiac might have spots on their new teeth with no enamel, delayed eruption of their teeth (either baby or adult), and multiple cavities.

Canker sores (also known as aphthous ulcers) occur in both adults and children with undiagnosed celiac disease (and in those already diagnosed who ingest gluten accidentally). These painful mouth sores frequently crop up on the inside of your lips in areas where you've had a very minor injury (such as a scratch from a sharp piece of food, a utensil, or your teeth). Once they start, they can take up to a week to subside. It's also not unusual to find celiac disease in a person who has periodontal disease or badly receding gums. In some cases, the gluten-free diet can help to reverse some of the damage that's been done.

Causes and Risk Factors of Celiac Disease

It's not entirely clear what causes celiac disease. In fact, most researchers believe multiple factors are involved, including your genes, your environment, and the foods you eat. You need some or even all of these factors to be present in order to develop celiac disease.

Common Causes

Celiac disease is an autoimmune disease in which gluten in your diet triggers your white blood cells to attack the tiny, finger-like projections called villi that line your small intestine and normally help you digest food. The lining is eroded until it's worn smooth. Without villi, you can't absorb vitamins, minerals, and other nutrients from food.

Your genes play a very strong role—if you don't have one of the two specific genes that have been linked to celiac disease, your odds of developing the condition are very low (although they are not zero; medical research has found people who have celiac but not those genes). However, because 30 percent of the population has one of the genes, and only 3 percent of the population with one or both of these genes develop celiac disease, genetics isn't the only factor.

To develop celiac disease, you must be eating gluten. When you have celiac disease, gluten spurs your immune system to attack your small intestine. Gluten is common in the Western-style diet, so it would be unusual to avoid it when not following a strict gluten-free diet.

Finally, for you to develop celiac disease, certain factors in your environment must help to cause it. It's these factors that aren't clear; some people can consume gluten every day for decades without a problem and then develop severe celiac disease symptoms very suddenly, while some young children exhibit celiac symptoms as soon as gluten-containing grains are introduced into their diets. Many women begin to experience celiac symptoms following pregnancy and birth, and other people find their symptoms begin following a seemingly unrelated illness or even following a stressful time in their life. There is also research into whether a virus might trigger the condition.

Besides having first-degree family members with celiac disease, risk factors include having lymphocytic colitis, Down syndrome, Turner syndrome, type 1 diabetes mellitus, and autoimmune (Hashimoto) thyroiditis, and Addison's disease.

Genetics

The two main genes for celiac disease are HLA-DQ2 and HLA-DQ8. About 96 percent of those diagnosed with celiac disease (by biopsy) have one or both of those genes. Certain subsets of the HLA-DQ2 gene can increase or decrease your risk. It's likely, too, that there are other genes involved that haven't yet been identified. Genes are inherited, and as a result celiac disease is seen to run in families. If you have a first-degree relative (parent, sibling, or child) with celiac disease you have a 5 percent to 22 percent chance of having celiac disease.

HLA-DQ2 is common among people with European heritage, seen in up to 40 percent of that population. HLA-DQ8 is most common in people from Central and South America but also appears in about 10 percent of the overall population. There's some evidence that carrying two copies of one of the genes (either DQ2 or DQ8) may increase your risk. You would have two copies if you inherited one copy from each parent.

Genetic testing for the genes associated with celiac disease is done by collecting cells from your mouth with a swab or by spitting into a vial. This can be done by your doctor, by specialized laboratories, or even by commercial genetic profile companies.

Lifestyle Risk Factors

Eating gluten is a necessary factor in developing celiac disease. Without gluten, the reaction that injures the villi doesn't happen. But you would have to grow up in an extremely cautious gluten-free household to have avoided gluten your entire life.

Gluten is found in wheat and some other grains. There is conflicting research as to whether the hybridized wheat of today has more gluten than wheat from a century ago. But wheat, gluten, and other gluten-containing grains are found in many processed foods, which may result in people having more exposure to gluten. One theory that's not correct is blaming the rise in celiac disease and non-celiac gluten sensitivity on genetically modified wheat. Since genetically-modified wheat isn't on the market anywhere, it can't be causing an increase.

There is ongoing research into whether feeding patterns in the first year of life make a difference in developing celiac disease. These studies have not found any effect associated with whether or not a child was breastfed and when gluten was first introduced to the diet. There is weak evidence that having a high amount of gluten at the time of weaning might increase the risk of celiac disease in children who have a high familial risk.

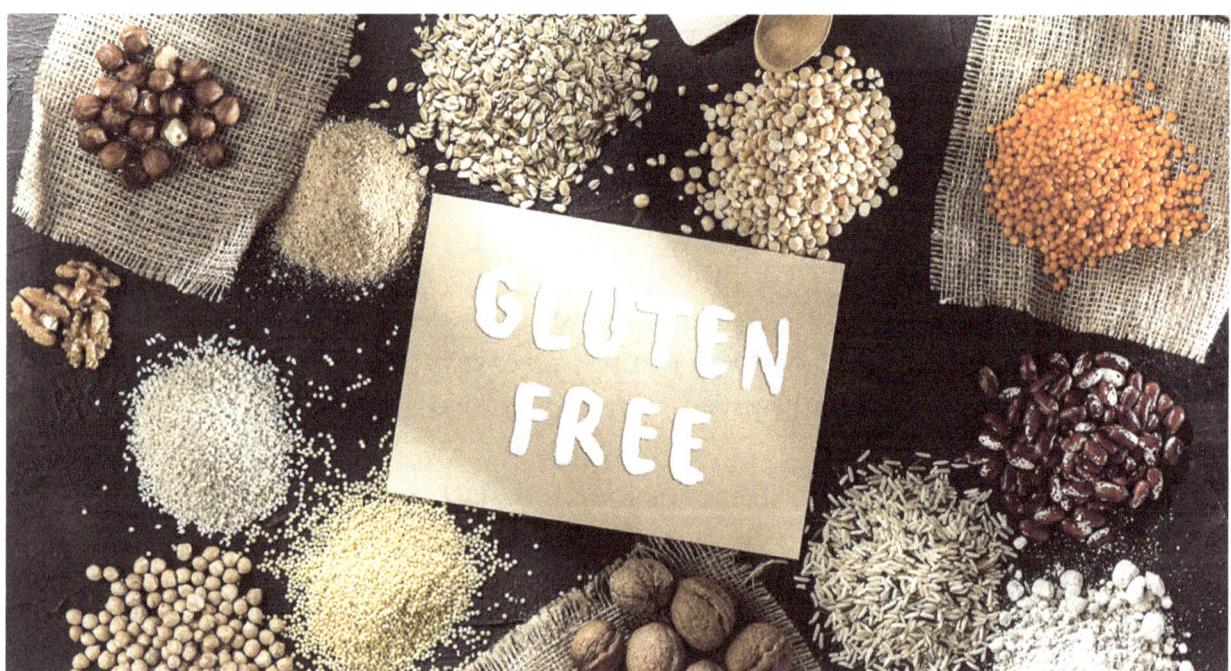

How Your Doctor Diagnoses Celiac Disease

The diagnosis of celiac disease is a fairly lengthy process. In most cases, you'll first have blood tests done, and then ultimately, will have a procedure known as an endoscopy, in which doctors look directly at your small intestine.1 In the best-case scenario, you'll have your answer within a few days or a week, but the diagnostic process can take much longer in some areas, especially where gastroenterologists (specialists in the digestive system) are in short supply.1 Here's what to expect from every stage of the process.

Self Checks/At-Home Testing

Some people go onto a gluten-free diet to see if it clears up their symptoms that might be associated with celiac disease. Whether or not this improves your symptoms, it should be followed up with diagnostic testing by your doctor.

There are at-home screening tests you can purchase for celiac disease. These use a finger-prick blood sample that you send to a laboratory, receiving the results in about a week.2 A home blood test should always be followed up with medical testing by a physician.

Important

You must be eating gluten for celiac disease testing to be accurate. If you are being tested for celiac disease, do not go gluten-free until all your testing is completed. Medical guidelines recommend celiac disease testing for relatives of those diagnosed with celiac disease since the condition runs in families. The familial risk is due to specific genes. Some people take advantage of consumer genetic testing, such as through 23andMe, to screen for celiac-related genes.3 This testing doesn't require being on a gluten-containing diet. It also only shows a risk of the disease, rather than markers of having celiac disease.

Labs and Tests

In most cases, celiac disease blood testing (which can be ordered by your primary care doctor) will be the first step toward a diagnosis. There are several blood tests commonly used to detect celiac disease, although many doctors will only request one or two of the tests. These tests look for various antibodies.4 If your body is undergoing an autoimmune reaction to gluten, one or more of these blood tests should come up positive. This indicates that further testing is needed to see if you truly have celiac disease.

However, it is possible for you to have negative blood test results and to still have celiac disease. Some people have a condition known as IgA deficiency that can cause false-negative results on some celiac disease blood tests. If you have this (there's yet another blood test that will look for it), you'll need different tests to screen for celiac disease.

In a few other cases, the blood test results simply don't reflect the amount of intestinal damage present. This also is known as a "false negative" test result. Therefore, if your blood tests are negative, but your symptoms and family medical history still indicate a strong possibility of celiac disease, you should talk to your physician about further testing.

Because the tests for celiac disease are looking specifically for signs of this small intestine damage, you must be eating gluten for the tests to be accurate. If you're not eating gluten-containing foods or not eating enough of them it's possible for the testing to come up negative, even if you actually do have celiac disease. Therefore, you should continue eating a normal diet, with gluten-containing foods several times a day, until all your testing is completed.

Of course, some people do go gluten-free before they decide to be tested for celiac disease. If you've already started following the gluten-free diet, you may want to consider what's called a "gluten challenge," in which you eat a set amount of gluten for some period of time, and then undergo testing for celiac disease. This tactic does carry some risks, though, and may not produce the results you want, so talk to your doctor about the potential risks and benefits.

Blood Tests for Celiac Disease

Genetic Testing

In some cases, your doctor may recommend genetic testing for celiac disease. Celiac disease is linked to two specific genes, which are passed down through families. Genetic tests can be done using a swab of your mouth or by drawing blood. The genetic test for celiac is the one test you can undergo regardless of whether you're currently eating gluten or not.

Genetic tests can't tell you if you actually have celiac disease for that, you'll need to undergo the blood tests and endoscopy described above. But genetic tests can tell you whether you have one of the genes you generally need to develop celiac disease.

If you don't have one of these two main genes, the odds of you having celiac disease are very slim, although some cases of celiac have been documented in people who don't carry either gene.

A positive genetic test for celiac disease doesn't mean you definitely have celiac disease—up to 40% of the population carries one of those genes, and the vast majority never develop celiac.7 However, it does mean you possibly can develop the condition. You'll need to discuss with your doctor your next steps if your celiac disease gene test comes back positive, especially if you have a family history of celiac disease.

How Celiac Disease Is Treated

There is no cure for celiac disease and the only treatment known to be effective is a gluten-free diet. Other therapies may be used if a gluten-free diet is unable to provide relief. Although celiac disease can cause deep frustration and anxiety, by working with your doctor and gastroenterologist, you should be more than able to manage your condition and live a full, productive life.

Home Remedies and Lifestyle

At present, a gluten-free diet is the only therapeutic approach able to control celiac disease. By removing the autoimmune trigger, namely gluten, the immune system will have no reason to react abnormally. Strict adherence to a gluten-free diet can help the intestines heal, resolve chronic symptoms, and reduce the risk to complications such as ulcers, bowel stricture, osteoporosis, and intestinal cancer.

Foods to Avoid

As simple as this may sound, a gluten-free diet can be cumbersome and difficult to maintain, particularly in areas where gluten-free food options are limited. It requires a fundamental change in how you approach eating, even if your current diet is healthy and balanced.

Cereal grains, the primary source of gluten, form a major part of the Western diet. To control celiac disease, you may need to avoid many, if not all, sources of gluten depending on your level of sensitivity to gluten and the stage of your disease. These include:

Wheat (including durum, einkorn, and emmer)

- Wheat germ
- Rye
- Barley
- Bulgur

- Couscous
- Farina
- Graham flour
- Kamut matzo
- Semolina
- Spelt
- Triticale

On top of that, you would need to avoid ingredients or packaged foods that contain or are derived from the above-listed grains. These may include:

- Bacon
- Baked goods
- Beer
- Bouillon cubes
- Bread
- Breakfast cereals
- Candies
- Canned baked beans
- Cold cuts
- Egg substitutes
- French fries (which are often dusted in flour)
- Gravy
- Hot dogs
- Ice cream
- Instant hot drinks
- Ketchup
- Malt flavoring
- Mayonnaise
- Meatballs
- Non-dairy creamer
- Oats or oat bran (if not certified gluten-free)
- Pasta
- Processed cheese
- Pudding and fruit filling
- Roasted nuts

- Salad dressings
- Sausage
- Seitan
- Soups
- Soy sauce
- Tabbouleh
- Veggie burgers
- Vodka
- Wheatgrass
- Wine coolers

In the United States, a product can be labeled "gluten-free" if it contains less than 20 parts per million (ppm) of gluten. While the threshold is usually low enough to avoid symptoms in most people living with the disease, there are some who will react to levels as low as five to 10 ppm.

People with extreme gluten sensitivity may also need to avoid certain non-food products that contain gluten, such as cosmetics, lip balms, shampoos, and non-adhesive stamps and envelopes.

Prescription and over-the-counter medications sometimes use wheat gluten as a binding agent. Talk to your gastroenterologist about the drugs you are taking so that substitutions can be made.

Vitamins and dietary supplements that contain wheat gluten must have "wheat" listed on the label.

Work with a Dietician

The best way to embark on a gluten-free diet is to work with a registered dietitian (RD) who is medically trained and certified in dietetics (as opposed to a nutritionist who may not be). The dietitian can work closely with your doctor to build a dietary strategy based on your medical results and lifestyle.

This is especially important since many Americans get their nutrients and daily fiber from fortified, gluten-containing products like cereal and bread. Working with a dietitian can help identify and prevent nutritional deficiencies that can arise from the loss of dietary gluten.

Because a gluten-free diet can be so challenging, particularly at the start, the dietitian will offer food substitutions to help ease you into the changes. You will also be offered dietary counseling so that you will be better able to:

Read and understand food labels

Understand where gluten is "hidden" in foods

Find the appropriate foods to eat in restaurants

Avoid accidental gluten cross-contamination in your home

Source gluten-free foods and non-food products online or at stores

Foods to Eat

As challenging as all of this may seem, a gluten-free diet is really not all that different from most healthy diets. In addition to avoiding packaged or processed foods, you would fill your plate with naturally wholesome gluten-free foods such as:

- Eggs
- Dairy including yogurt, butter, and non-processed cheeses (but check the label of flavored dairy products)
- Fruits and vegetables including most which are canned or dried
- Grains including rice, quinoa, corn, millet, tapioca, buckwheat, amaranth, arrowroot, teff, and gluten-free oats
- Legumes like beans, lentils, peas, peanuts
- Meat, poultry, and fish (not breaded or battered)
- Non-gluten starches including potato flour, corn flour, chickpea flour, soy flour, almond meal/flour, coconut flour, and

tapioca flour
- Nuts and seeds
- Soy foods like tofu, tempeh, and edamame
- Tamari (a good substitute for soy sauce)
- Vegetable oils (preferably monounsaturated or polyunsaturated)
- Prepared foods certified gluten-free are increasingly available on grocery store shelves, including bread, baked goods, frozen meals, and gluten-free meal kits.

An Overview of the Gluten-Free Diet

Avoiding Accidental Gluten Exposure

Managing celiac disease involves more than just a change in diet; it requires a change in lifestyle and the support of the people around you. This is not always easy.

Trying to maintain two separate diets in a family can not only be time-consuming but may also expose you to gluten cross-contamination. On the other hand, placing a child without celiac disease on a gluten-free diet can be unhealthy.

It is important, therefore, to achieve "buy-in" from those around you. Even loved ones with the best of intentions may not understand celiac disease and turn off the second you mention the words "gluten-free." By educating friends and family members, you will able to maintain a gluten-free lifestyle and experience less resistance from those around you.

There are other tips to help avoid gluten exposure at home or in restaurants:

Keep gluten-free and gluten-containing foods separate in sealed containers and in separate drawers or cabinets.

Clean cooking surfaces and food storage areas.

Wash dishes, utensils, and food preparation equipment thoroughly.

Avoid wood utensils or cutting boards that can absorb food and potentiate cross-contamination.

Speak to your child's teachers and lunch staff if he or she has celiac disease so that accidents can be avoided and special accommodations can be made.

Check restaurant menus online before eating out to be sure there are food items you can eat.

Call the restaurant in advance to inform them about your health concerns and dietary needs.

Book early or late when a restaurant is less busy and better able to accommodate your special requests.

How To Recover From Accidental Gluten Exposure

Prescriptions

A gluten-free diet may be all that is needed to control celiac disease symptoms and prevent flares. But, for some people, this may not be enough. In fact, according to a 2015 study in the journal Digestive Diseases, between 1% and 2% of people with celiac disease will not respond to a gluten-free diet.

The condition, referred to as refractory celiac disease, is rare but serious and can significantly increase the risk of a type of cancer known as T-cell lymphoma. To avoid this, your doctor may prescribe medications that actively suppress the immune system and, with it, the autoimmune response.

Drug treatments are only indicated if you have had villous atrophy and malabsorption symptoms for at least six to 12 months despite strict adherence to a gluten-free diet.

The first-line drug of choice is a class of steroids known as a glucocorticoid. Prednisolone and budesonide are the two oral glucocorticoids mostly commonly prescribed.

While effective at alleviating symptoms, glucocorticoids only appear to reverse intestinal damage in around 33% of patients, according to a 2014 review in Therapeutic Advances in Chronic Diseases.2 Glucocorticoids can also mask the signs of the intestinal lymphoma.

Other pharmaceutical options include:

Asacol (mesalamine), an oral nonsteroidal anti-inflammatory drug (NSAID) sometimes used in people with Crohn's disease

Cyclosporine, an oral disease-modifying antirheumatic drug (DMARD) used to treat a variety of autoimmune disorders

Imuran (azathioprine), an oral immunosuppressive drug traditionally used in organ transplant recipients

Remicade (infliximab), an injectable biologic drug that blocks the chemical processes that lead to inflammation

In rare cases when T-cell lymphoma is diagnosed, combination chemotherapy would be used. The mainstay of treatment is CHOP therapy (an anagram referring to the drugs cyclophosphamide, doxorubicin, vincristine, and prednisone).

Other promising drugs in the developmental pipeline including larazotide acetate (a potent digestive enzyme that breaks down dietary gluten) and BL-7010 (a high-density polymer that binds to gluten so that it cannot be absorbed).

Surgeries and Specialist-Driven Procedures

In addition to steroids, people with refractory celiac disease may be placed on an elemental diet, a type of liquid diet that is more readily absorbed than solid foods. Total parenteral nutrition (TPN), in which nutrients are delivered through a vein, may be recommended for those with extreme weight loss who are unable to eat.

Surgery

Surgery is not used to treat celiac disease per se but rather to treat complications of the disease, including bowel obstruction, perforation, hemorrhage, and malignancy (cancer).

According to a 2015 study in American Surgery, which evaluated the medical records of 512 adults with celiac disease for 22 years, no less than 11% underwent abdominal surgery as a direct result of the disease.

In people with T-cell lymphoma, surgery may be used in advance of chemotherapy to prevent the perforation of vulnerable tissues.

Autologous stem cell transplant in which stems cells are harvested from your body prior to chemotherapy and returned to you afterward have been used successfully to treat intestinal lymphoma in people with refractory celiac disease.

Complementary Alternative Medicine (CAM

By most accounts, a gluten-free diet is considered the most "natural" approach to celiac disease possible. With that being said, complementary and alternative practitioners believe that there are other ways to control the symptoms of celiac disease and/or better tolerate a gluten-free diet.

Peppermint Oil

Peppermint oil has antispasmodic effects that may help ease intestinal cramping and spasms. Research from the University of South Alabama reported that a sustained-release peppermint oil capsule was twice as effective in alleviating irritable bowel syndrome (IBS) than a placebo. Whether the same would occur with celiac disease has yet to be confirmed. Peppermint oil taken directly by mouth may cause heartburn and stomach upset. Enteric-coated peppermint capsules are less likely to cause harm. Excessive doses of peppermint oil can be toxic.

Slippery Elm Powder

Slippery elm powder is derived from the bark of the slippery elm. Some people believe that it can protect the intestines by creating a mucus-like coating as it is digested. A 2010 study in the Journal of Alternative and Complementary Medicine reported that slippery elm powder as able to ease symptoms of constipation-dominant irritable bowel syndrome (IBS-C).

The same effect may be useful in treating constipation that commonly occurs with a gluten-free diet. There is no evidence thus far that slippery elm powder can treat symptoms of celiac disease itself.

Coping With Celiac Disease

Depression, anxiety, and fatigue are three of the most common symptoms reported by those coping with celiac disease. The emotional component of coping with celiac disease can be perplexing, particularly for those who have not experienced the disease first-hand. Because celiac disease is a long-term autoimmune disorder, there are multiple issues at play; for example, malabsorption—a common symptom of celiac disease—is thought to play a part in depression.

Changing to a gluten-free diet to treat celiac disease is not only a practical concern but also an emotional one. Food is part of just about every major life event, including weddings, funerals, birthdays, graduations, holidays, and everyday celebrations of getting a new job or going on a date night. For those with celiac disease, it encompasses a lot more than just what's on the menu.

Emotional

There are several factors involved when it comes to emotionally coping with celiac disease. For example, there may be the sadness (emotional response) of knowing that you must give up many of the foods that you have enjoyed for years. Then there is the psychological impact. For example, depression and anxiety are not considered emotions, but certainly have emotional attributes. Most people feel sad when they are depressed and experience fear when they have anxiety. So, when considering how to cope with celiac disease, it's important to bear in mind a person's emotional and psychological reactions.

Coping With Frustration

In addition to the sadness surrounding not being able to eat favorite (and familiar) foods, many people with celiac disease go through an initial phase of frustration. Finding your way through the grocery store the first several times when planning a gluten-free diet can be insurmountably aggravating.

It's not uncommon to end up spending several hours at the store, reading labels and making food choices, only to end up leaving with far fewer groceries than you intended to purchase.

The frustration of starting a new diet usually improves with time, but it can help to buddy up with someone who knows the ropes; perhaps consider shopping with a person who is an experienced gluten-free shopper (particularly during the initial shopping trip).

Coping With Psychological Aspects

Emotional symptoms (such as anger, sadness, and more) may be linked to coping with a diagnosis of a major illness that will require a significant lifestyle change. But symptoms could also be a direct result of a psychological condition—such as depression— which can result from common physical symptoms of celiac disease (such as malabsorption and chronic inflammation).

Studies have shown a possible link between abnormal brain function and malabsorption of nutrients. The risk of becoming depressed is 1.8 times greater when a person has celiac disease.

Research has shown that there can be several physiological factors linked with emotional symptoms involved when a person has celiac disease, including:

Vitamin deficiency from malabsorption, particularly Vitamins D, K, B, B6, B12, iron, calcium, and folate

Biochemical imbalance in the brain due to the inability to produce enough tryptophan (needed for the production of serotonin, dopamine, and other neurotransmitters)

Toxins (that build up due to leaky gut syndrome and other physiological symptoms of celiac disease)

Long-term impact on organs which may develop primary disease. For example, up to 80% of those with celiac disease who also have depression are diagnosed with thyroid disease

Although eating a gluten-free diet can begin to alleviate many symptoms of celiac disease within a few weeks (or even a few days in some instances), depression, anxiety, and fatigue may linger. In fact, these symptoms may not subside for a year, or even longer. This may be due to a combination of different factors including:

Difficulty adjusting to changes in the new diet and lifestyle

Feelings of loss linked to no longer being able to indulge in certain foods or feeling like an outsider when visiting restaurants, engaging in social get-togethers (where food is being served) and more

Lack of adequate nutrients (it takes time—sometimes up to a year or even longer—for the body to adjust and get back to normal, once the gut begins to heal and nutrients are being absorbed again)

Having a chronic negative thinking pattern (caused by depression, anxiety, or other factors)

Sometimes people get into a rut. Having celiac-linked depression or anxiety can result in long-term negative thinking. Many people with celiac disease find that getting involved in some type of mindfulness practice, such as mindfulness-based stress reduction (MBSR), can really help break old habits. Be sure to look for an instructor who is certified, and preferably one who has worked with people who have depression and anxiety, and/or with those diagnosed with celiac disease.

Study

In a 2015 review of the literature, study authors discovered that "anxiety, depression, and fatigue are common complaints in patients with untreated celiac disease and contribute to lower quality of life." Although many of these symptoms subside once treatment starts, these symptoms often impact a person's adherence to treatment.4 The study authors concluded that "healthcare professionals should be aware of the ongoing psychological burden of celiac disease in order to support patients with this disease." The Celiac Foundation reports that a wide range of emotional and behavioral symptoms of celiac disease can occur, these may include:

Lack of experiencing pleasure in life

Socially withdrawing

Losing interest in hobbies or activities once enjoyed

Having mood swings

Experiencing unusually low energy levels

Feeling aggressive or angry much of the time

A change in eating (loss or an increase in appetite)

A change in sleeping patterns (sleeping more or insomnia)

Feelings of extreme guilt or worthlessness

Having racing thoughts or feeling agitation

Hearing voices

Believing others are planning against you

These symptoms may be warning signs that a person needs to seek mental health treatment, particularly when experiencing any type of suicidal thoughts, or thoughts of harming self or others.

Keep in mind that many of these feelings are common in people with celiac disease, particularly when the disorder is newly diagnosed or untreated. It's important to seek help (including professional help, support groups, or more) when needed, but at the same time, avoid any type of self-blame.

Coping With Emotions When You're Newly Gluten-Free

Physical

Physical aspects that can help lessen emotional symptoms and enable people to cope more effectively with celiac disease may include:

Long-term adherence to the gluten-free diet (which often alleviates symptoms)

Regular exercise (to help improve mood, and boost energy levels) Approximately 5 minutes of exercise each day can start to alleviate stress and anxiety5

For some people, exercise, along with other tools, helps depression. Many people combine a regular workout with involvement in support groups, meditation practice, mindfulness practice, medication, and more.

Consult your primary provider before starting any type of physical exercise routine.

Diet

A gluten-free diet is the primary treatment modality for celiac disease.

One reason depression may occur in people with celiac disease is due to a lack of proper absorption of vitamins such as vitamin B. Symptoms may continue even after treatment has started to heal the gut (where absorption of nutrients occurs). A simple vitamin supplement may provide adequate nutrients and alleviate symptoms.

Common supplements given for celiac disease include:

Iron

Calcium

Zinc

Vitamin D

Niacin and folate (B vitamins)

Magnesium

It's important to consult with your health care provider before taking any type of vitamin or supplement, and be sure to select a gluten-free product. Keep in mind that when taking a multivitamin, the dose should never exceed the 100% daily value for vitamins and minerals.3

An Overview of the Gluten-Free Diet

After a diagnosis of celiac disease, you will need to go on a gluten-free diet. It helps to start with understanding exactly what gluten is so you can begin to identify what to eliminate.

Gluten is in many foods (including many in which you wouldn't expect to find it) and it's extremely difficult to avoid. In fact, the learning curve on a gluten-free diet is equal to or greater than the learning curves on almost any other type of diet. You will get the hang of it eventually, but you'll learn more about food labeling and ingredient names than you ever thought you would need to know in the process.

You'll also make mistakes as you learn how to eat gluten-free. They're inevitable, so don't beat yourself up over them—even if your body beats you up because of them. Even when you've been eating gluten-free for a decade or more, you'll probably still make mistakes, although they likely won't be too severe.

What Is Gluten

The gluten you need to avoid is a protein found in grains like wheat, barley, and rye. So, any food that contains wheat, barley, and rye thus contains gluten, such as bread, pasta, cakes, cookies, and most cereal. Gluten-containing grains are commonly used in foods because they have characteristics that are prized by food manufacturers. For example, wheat bread gets its distinctive, pleasing elasticity and texture from gluten, while cakes and pasta stick together instead of crumbling because of the gluten protein.

However, bread, cereal, and pasta represent only the tip of the gluten iceberg—gluten is an ingredient in many, possibly even the majority of, processed food products. In certain soups, gluten grains act as thickeners, allowing manufacturers and cooks at home to use less expensive ingredients such as cream. Barley malt, meanwhile, is frequently used as a sweetener in candy and cookies. And in beer and some forms of liquor, gluten grains are fermented to make alcoholic brews.

There are some foods that always contain gluten, such as conventional bread products and pasta. But avoiding these just isn't enough if you're following a gluten-free diet. You need to eliminate every scrap of gluten even the ingredients that are hidden.

Why Eat Gluten-Free

Most people who follow a gluten-free diet do so because they're using it to treat a specific health condition. The best-known health condition that responds to a gluten-free diet is celiac disease. When those with celiac disease consume wheat, barley, or rye, the gluten in the grain triggers the immune system to attack the lining of the small intestine. This triggers celiac disease symptoms and can lead to malnutrition, anemia, osteoporosis, and many other potentially serious health consequences.

People with celiac disease must be gluten-free for life in order to alleviate symptoms and significantly reduce the risk of related conditions. Even tiny amounts of gluten can keep immune systems in overdrive and prevent intestines from healing.

Doctors recommend that people not start eating gluten-free before being tested for celiac disease. That's because you need to be consuming gluten for celiac disease testing to be accurate.1 It can be important to know for sure whether you have celiac so that you can watch for related health conditions that might occur.

What Foods Contain Gluten

To eat gluten-free, you'll need to avoid everything that contains wheat, barley, and rye. Getting rid of the obvious items bread, pasta, crackers, and cookies—should be pretty easy (although it can be rough emotionally to let go of your favorite foods, even if you're replacing them with gluten-free substitutes).

The problem is that gluten can hide under various ingredients on a food label. Do you have a can of soup in your cupboard that contains "starch"? That starch might contain gluten. What about that candy with "natural flavors"? Potential gluten there, too. It's seemingly everywhere and you'll need to figure out where it hides in order to avoid it.

The U.S. Food and Drug Administration (FDA) does not require disclosure of gluten on food labels, although manufacturers can disclose it voluntarily under the FDA's gluten-free labeling rules.

To use the FDA's "gluten-free" label, a food must not have any type of wheat, rye, barley, or crossbreeds of those grains. The food can't use an ingredient derived from those grains unless it has been processed to remove gluten to less than 20 parts per million (ppm).

Many companies do choose to make it easy for people to identify their gluten-free products without looking at the ingredients. They'll use bold labeling that states "gluten-free" or a symbol that means "gluten-free." The growing popularity of the diet has ensured that all kinds of gluten-free products can be found in many mainstream grocery stores. You can also purchase foods specifically certified gluten-free by an independent organization.

Other manufacturers, like Kraft Foods and Con Agra Foods, have policies of always disclosing ingredients that contain gluten in their food labels. In those cases, a gluten-containing starch would be labeled in the ingredients list as "starch (wheat)," while a gluten-containing natural flavor might read "flavoring (barley)." However, foods with no gluten ingredients aren't necessarily gluten-free since they could be subject to gluten cross-contamination in processing.

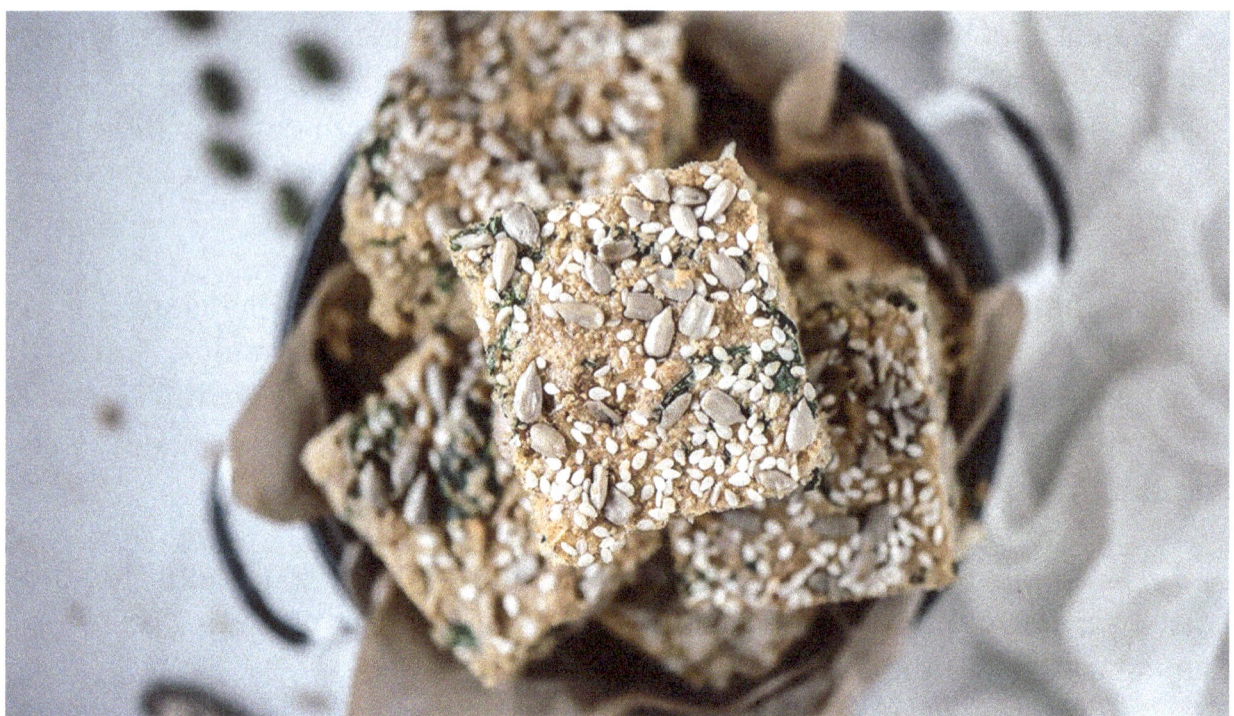

How to Start a Gluten-Free Diet

Given all of this, you might think eating gluten-free seems a bit intimidating. But you can actually eat gluten-free without reading a single food label, just stick entirely to naturally gluten-free whole foods such as fresh fruits, vegetables, meats, poultry, and fish.

This, in fact, is the best way to start a gluten-free diet because it prevents you from making rookie mistakes while your body adjusts. This approach will also help you isolate any symptoms later on when you've added in more foods. Furthermore, it may help you consume more needed nutrients since packaged goods have less of those all-important vitamins and minerals than fresh, whole foods.

There's actually quite a long list of reliably and safely gluten-free foods. If you're shopping in the produce section, for example, all the fresh fruits and vegetables are safe to consume on a gluten-free diet (although anything that comes pre-packaged might not be). In the meat section, stick to beef, poultry, pork, and seafood that doesn't contain marinades or other added ingredients. Basically, as long as it's plain, it's safe.

Rice and quinoa are both good choices as a starch to add to your diet—just be certain to buy plain varieties with no added ingredients. Potatoes can also be a good choice, although you'll need to watch how they're prepared. Dessert can be a bit tricky since many of the classic go-to's contain gluten (think pie, cookies, and cakes). Ice cream may be a good choice—unless you're lactose intolerant, a common problem in those with celiac disease. Be especially careful to stick to an ice cream brand and flavor that's considered gluten-free (yes, ice cream can contain gluten).

Avoid Trace Amounts

You may be surprised to find that once you've started eating gluten-free, your body will react to even tiny amounts of gluten with a replay of old symptoms or even new ones you weren't expecting. Such symptoms may include digestive upset and fatigue. Unfortunately, this is pretty common after a gluten exposure and can take several days, or more, to feel like yourself again.

Also, some people are just more sensitive to gluten cross-contamination than others. Unfortunately, this means they have to be extra careful. Regardless of where you wind up falling on the sensitivity scale, you'll need to do some homework when you first go gluten-free to minimize the chance of an accidental glutening. Specifically, you'll need to:

Decide whether to share a kitchen with household members who eat gluten and (if the decision is yes) set up that shared kitchen in a way that prevents you from getting sick.Banish gluten foods and ingredients from your kitchen (or from the part of the kitchen you'll be using if you're planning a shared kitchen).

Replace kitchen tools since they're likely to harbor gluten grain residue (even though you've scrubbed them thoroughly).

Make the rest of your home gluten-free, including your bathroom (shampoo, conditioner, toothpaste, and makeup), your workshop (drywall and craft supplies can contain gluten), and your medicine cabinet.

Exercise some serious caution when dining out and eating food prepared by a friend or family member.

There are ways to make the process of going gluten-free easier. You can, for example, download a smartphone app to help you identify products and restaurants that cater to those who are gluten-free. You can also check in with your favorite grocery store to see if it maintains lists of gluten-free products or labels the products on their shelves. And, you can bring your own food to gatherings where you don't think the food provided will be gluten-free enough for you.

How to Go Gluten-Free

Clean Out Your Kitchen

Before you can start the gluten-free diet, you need to clean out your kitchen and get rid of everything you no longer can eat. Learn the foods that contain gluten. They include:

- most breads, crackers, cookies, and snack foods
- most mixes
- most pasta
- many frozen food products
- many canned soups
- some ice creams

This isn't an exhaustive list, unfortunately; gluten appears in many places you wouldn't expect. If in doubt, throw it out: Give away or dispose of everything, especially wheat flour and baking mixes. When doing so, you'll need to be careful not to breathe any airborne flour, which can make you sick.

You'll also need to replace any open condiments since they're likely to have been cross-contaminated with gluten (when someone touches the tip of a squeeze bottle to bread or sticks a used sandwich knife in a jar, the bottle or jar could make you sick). The same goes for spices you've used in baking since those likely have been cross-contaminated by wheat flour.

Donate unopened gluten-containing packages, jars, and cans to a food bank or hand them over to a friend. Alternatively, if you're planning on sharing a kitchen with family members or housemates who don't eat gluten-free, you'll need to segregate those products.

Since it's possible to get symptoms from the tiniest morsel of gluten, you'll need a new toaster. You'll also need new plastic and wooden utensils and non-stick pans if you use them. Replace all these kitchen tools when you go gluten-free since they can't be cleaned thoroughly enough to keep you safe.

For some people, this is a difficult, emotional process—you may find yourself mourning the foods you used to enjoy. If that's the case, it can help to focus on the positive effect the gluten-free diet will have on your health. Also, if you can afford it, use this opportunity to treat yourself to a new kitchen tool you've been coveting.

Start With Fresh Produce and Meats

Many people think they simply need to drop wheat from their diets—or even just bread—in order to go gluten-free. But it's unfortunately a lot more complicated than that. As you no doubt learned from cleaning out your kitchen, gluten appears in foods ranging from soups to sauces, and it's not always obvious from the ingredients.

There are many, many foods you can eat on the list of gluten-free foods. But by far the best way to avoid making common mistakes when first going gluten-free is to limit your diet to unprocessed foods at first. Unprocessed foods are products you find in the supermarket that don't have ingredients lists printed on their labels; for example, fresh fruits and vegetables and fresh meat, poultry, and fish are examples of unprocessed foods.

On an unprocessed food diet, you can eat:

- fresh fruit
- fresh vegetables
- beef (only from the meat counter and unseasoned)
- chicken (only from the meat counter and unseasoned)
- pork (only from the meat counter and unseasoned)
- fish (only from the fish counter and unseasoned)
- milk, yogurt, and cheese
- eggs

To follow an unprocessed foods diet, shop around the edges of the supermarket, in the fresh produce and meat departments. If you can handle dairy products (many people with celiac disease have lactose intolerance, at least at first), you also can add dairy products. Eat as simply as you can, using only fresh herbs, salt, and pepper to season your foods.

The safest grain to add to your diet is plain rice Lundberg Family Farms produces rice that's certified gluten-free. Try grains such as corn in moderation, if at all, and don't introduce packaged foods—including those labeled "gluten-free" until you have a better feel for the diet and how it affects your system.

Expand to Include Gluten-Free Labeled Products

Once you've mastered the basics, foods clearly labeled "gluten-free" represent the best way to start expanding your gluten-free diet. Manufacturers aren't required to label foods "gluten-free," but many do. When you're still learning how to stay gluten-free, you shouldn't count on your ability to read labels—stick with products that market to the gluten-free community. You won't be limited in your selection. On supermarket shelves, you'll find gluten-free versions of practically everything you want, including:

- gluten-free bread
- gluten-free pizza
- gluten-free frozen waffles
- gluten-free beer
- gluten-free ice cream
- gluten-free yogurt
- gluten-free soup
- gluten-free candy

Be careful not to go overboard with the gluten-free-labeled products, since many people find they experience renewed gluten symptoms when they eat too much of these products. In some cases, symptoms could result from unhealed damage in your intestines. However, in most instances, the culprit is the tiny amounts of gluten still present in the "gluten-free"-labeled foods.

If you begin adding gluten-free-labeled foods to your diet but then start experiencing renewed (or even new) symptoms, or if you just don't feel particularly well, cut back on these products, especially anything you've added recently.

Learn to Read Food Labels

To really expand your diet and to figure out which of your old favorites you might be able to include—you'll need to learn to find gluten on food labels.

In fact, you'll probably become a bit of a detective, learning to search for the meaning of various terms you'll find on different products. You'll also get quite an education on the different ingredients that make up processed foods (some of them unpronounceable).

For example, terms that always mean "gluten" can include:

flour

triticum (the technical name for wheat)

hordeum (the technical name for barley)

spelt (a type of wheat)

Meanwhile, terms that almost always mean "gluten" can include:

malt (likely barley malt)

pasta (wheat unless otherwise specified)

Terms that may mean "gluten" can include:

vegetable protein (most often wheat or soy)

dextrin and maltodextrin (can be made from wheat, although that's not common in the U.S.)

Just remember: Manufacturers can label something "gluten-free," but food labeling laws do not require disclosure of gluten-containing ingredients on food labels. If something has no obvious gluten ingredients listed but doesn't carry a "gluten-free" label, it might contain barley or rye, or be subject to gluten cross-contamination at the food processing facility.

In addition, keep in mind that wheat-free does not equal gluten-free, so don't be fooled by foods labeled "wheat-free" — they're probably not safe.

You might want to consider getting one of the various gluten-free apps on the market to help guide your choices on processed food products, ingredients, and restaurants. Several apps provide lists of gluten-free products you can access while you are in the grocery store. A subscription-based app lets you scan a product's UPC code to determine if it's gluten-free or not.

Make Your Home Gluten-Free

You'd probably think you should focus on making your kitchen gluten-free... and you'd be right, at least at first. But as you get more skilled in following the gluten-free diet, you should consider removing sources of gluten that lurk elsewhere in your home.

For example, many hair products contain gluten. If you've ever gotten shampoo in your mouth in the shower, or if you touch your hair and then your mouth, you should consider getting gluten-free shampoo and other hair products. Also, check out your toothpaste and make sure it's on the list of gluten-free toothpaste options.

Making your bathroom and medicine cabinet gluten-free can be challenging, as well. Cosmetics and prescription medications also frequently contain gluten and can cause major symptoms if you're not careful. Here are some resources: Even art supplies and common household building materials, such as drywall and spackling compound, can contain gluten. Therefore, you should stick with gluten-free craft supplies.

Learn to Eat Out Gluten-Free

Until you feel confident following the gluten-free diet and ideally until any symptoms have largely disappeared you should stay far away from restaurants. That's because restaurants (and especially fast food restaurants) are a major risk for gluten cross-contamination. It's common for even experienced gluten-free dieters to inadvertently consume gluten when they eat out at restaurants. Still, no one wants to eat at home forever. Once you have a better idea of how to eat gluten-free and where gluten can hide, restaurant dining won't present as much of a challenge.

When you first try dining out gluten-free, be aware that many servers and even some chefs aren't very familiar with the gluten-free diet, and mistakes are (sadly) pretty common. Follow these tips to stay safe:

Stick with a restaurant (or a chain) that features a gluten-free menu, since restaurants with gluten-free menus are more likely to have spent time on staff education.

Discuss your needs with your server, the chef, or a manager.

Use gluten-free restaurant apps to find the best options.

Consider ethnic restaurants with gluten-free-friendly cuisines.

Be careful letting your guard down, even in a restaurant that has served you successfully before. Gluten-free restaurant cards can help you talk to restaurant staff about what to do and what to avoid doing.

Socialize ... But Bring Your Own Food

Once you go gluten-free, it's likely that friends and relatives may try to cook for you. Don't let them—realistically, unless you trust that person to avoid all gluten ingredients and cross contamination (e.g., unless they're also eating gluten-free or they hold professional chef or dietitian credentials), you're better off bringing your own food to social events. As you know by now, this diet has a ridiculously steep learning curve—it's not something a friend can master overnight, no matter how much that person wants to do so, and how hard they're likely to try.

Bringing your own food to gatherings allows you to focus on the company, as opposed to constantly worrying about getting sick. You'll be more relaxed (not constantly on guard against risks) and your friends won't be concerned about making you ill.

If you want, bring a dish to share. If you do this, though, fill your plate first, since cross contamination from other guests can be a risk (most people wouldn't think twice about using a spoon from the bread crumb-covered casserole in your safe vegetable dish).

Holidays can be particularly tricky emotionally when you're gluten-free. To cope with them, always make sure you have something with you that's both gluten-free and delicious. Don't be afraid to treat yourself—you shouldn't be deprived when everyone around you is enjoying good food.

Know That You'll Make Mistakes (and Learn From Them)

You'll absolutely make mistakes (and potentially get sick from them) as you learn to navigate the gluten-free diet. Your symptoms may return for a day, or even for a week or more in the worst cases. Unfortunately, once you go gluten-free, your body will be primed to make a big deal out of any little bit of gluten you consume. Most people (although not all) find they react badly to small amounts of cross-contamination.

It will take some time—months, probably—to learn your individual level of tolerance for gluten cross contamination, and what you can eat without getting symptoms.

It's tempting to beat yourself up for those mistakes mentally—especially if you're miserable physically. But if you can manage it, try to view them as a learning opportunity, and focus on avoiding making that same mistake twice.

Although there's no quick fix for the sickness you feel after accidentally eating gluten, there are some steps you can take to feel a little better:

Try to rest as much as possible.

Eat bland, safe foods such as rice.

Understand that you may experience some brain fog, and plan accordingly.

Gluten-Free Diet Benefits

1. May Ease Digestive Symptoms

Digestive issues like bloating, gas and diarrhea are some of the hallmark symptoms of gluten sensitivity, along with other side effects like fatigue and mood changes. Additionally, some of the typical symptoms for celiac disease include nausea, vomiting, flatulence and diarrhea. If you experience any of these issues after eating foods with gluten, cutting them out of your diet could significantly help reduce your symptoms.

A study in the American Journal of Gastroenterology looked at the effects of gluten on adults with non-celiac gluten sensitivity. After eating gluten daily for six weeks, participants reported a worsening of symptoms like poor stool consistency, pain, bloating and fatigue. If you regularly experience adverse digestive side effects after eating gluten-containing foods, consider an elimination diet to determine if a gluten-free diet could help provide long-term relief.

2. Can Provide Extra Energy

Some people report feeling tired or sluggish after eating foods with gluten. If this is the case for you, a gluten-free diet plan could provide some extra energy and prevent the brain fog and fatigue that may come from eating gluten. Celiac disease can also cause nutrient malabsorption, which could also be at the root of fatigue. For individuals who suffer these symptoms, eating gluten can trigger an immune response that causes your immune cells to attack the lining of the small intestine. Over time, the damage caused to the lining can impair the absorption of certain nutrients, making it difficult to get the proper nutrients needed to maintain energy levels. In particular, reduced levels of iron, folate, vitamin B12, vitamin D, zinc and magnesium are all often seen in patients not on a proper celiac disease diet.

Iron deficiency is especially common in those with celiac disease. This causes iron deficiency anemia, a condition that is characterized by a lack of healthy red blood cells, resulting in fatigue, lightheadedness and low energy.

If this is the case for you, removing gluten from your diet could help increase your energy levels and prevent the drained, sluggish feeling that can accompany gluten consumption. Remember to fill your gluten-free diet with plenty of nutrient-dense foods to close any nutritional gaps and keep energy levels up.

3. Could Benefit Children with Autism

Autism is a developmental disorder that causes impairments in communication and social interaction. Although autism affects people of all ages, most cases are identified within the first two years of life.

Traditional treatment for autism includes the use of different types of specialized therapy along with medications. However, promising new research has shown that eliminating gluten from the diet could help reduce symptoms of autism in children when used alone or in conjunction with conventional treatment methods.

A study in Nutritional Neuroscience, for example, found that strict adherence to a gluten-free, casein-free diet led to improvements in autism behaviors, physiological symptoms and social behaviors, according to parents.

Another study out of Iran reported that a gluten-free diet decreased gastrointestinal symptoms and significantly decreased behavioral disorders in children with autism.

Other autism natural treatments include using supplements like fish oil, digestive enzymes and probiotics, along with a healthy diet high of additive-free, unprocessed foods.

4. Can Decrease Inflammation

When those with celiac disease continue to consume gluten, it can contribute to widespread inflammation in the body over time. Inflammation is a normal immune response, but chronic inflammation may be linked to the development of chronic diseases like heart disease and cancer.

If you have celiac disease, a gluten-free diet could help you avoid inflammation and prevent harmful health consequences that could occur as a result.

One animal study noted that gluten intake shifted the balance of inflammatory immune cells in mice, causing an increase in markers of inflammation. Conversely, another animal study found that following a gluten-free diet improved levels of inflammatory markers in mice. However, more studies on humans are needed to determine whether a gluten-free diet can help reduce inflammation in humans, including those with and without celiac disease.

5. Promotes Fat Loss

In addition to reducing symptoms like digestive issues and fatigue, some research has also found that following a gluten-free diet may help promote fat loss. A 2013 animal study reported that mice given a gluten-free diet showed reductions in body weight and fat, even without any changes in food intake. They also had increases in specific receptors and enzymes that enhance the breakdown of fat

Another animal study in the International Journal of Obesity found that eating wheat gluten increased weight gain by decreasing the energy expenditure of fat tissue. Still, it remains unclear whether this same effect may be true for humans. More studies are needed focusing on the effects of gluten on body weight and body fat on humans specifically.

6. Improves Symptoms of Irritable Bowel Syndrome

Irritable bowel syndrome, or IBS, is an intestinal disorder that causes digestive symptoms like bloating, gas, constipation and diarrhea. A low-FODMAP, IBS diet is often recommended as a first-line defense against

IBS. This is a diet low in short-chain carbohydrates, which are not digested but instead fermented by the bacteria in the gut. Reducing your intake of these foods could help sidestep some of the negative symptoms of IBS.

Gluten-containing grains contain oligosaccharides, a type of short-chain carbohydrate that is easily fermentable in the gut, and are restricted on a low-FODMAP diet.

A study in the journal Gastroenterology compared the effects of a gluten-free and gluten-containing diet on participants with diarrhea-predominant IBS. Interestingly, researchers found that those eating gluten had increased bowel frequency and intestinal permeability (or leaky gut) compared to those on a gluten-free diet.

Makeup Brands That Offer Gluten-Free Options

Many of us with celiac disease and non-celiac gluten sensitivity find we feel better when our makeup is gluten-free. However, sleuthing out ingredients in makeup products—and then deciphering their chemical names to determine if they actually contain the protein gluten or not—is no small task. Below, you'll find a list of cosmetics companies and what they say about their gluten-free status, but first, why you should be concerned about makeup even though it's not something you eat.

Should I Buy Gluten-Free Makeup

As you probably know, your reaction to gluten stems from your digestive tract, not from your skin. In fact, the gluten protein is too large to be absorbed through your skin.

Therefore, makeup and skin care products (such as moisturizers) that you use on your skin but don't ingest shouldn't in theory be an issue unless you're using them on your lips. That's what many experts on celiac and gluten sensitivity will tell you.

It's difficult or impossible, though, to apply makeup or other skin care products without risking ingesting a tiny bit, either as you're spreading the product on your face, or later because you got some on your hands or under your fingernails and didn't wash it off thoroughly enough.

How many times have you noticed that weird, sometimes metallic, often fragrance-y makeup taste in your mouth? If you use skin care products every day, I'll bet you notice it fairly often. And that's the problem, in a nutshell.

Skin Conditions That Might Be a Sign of a Gluten Allergy

It Only Takes a Little Tiny Bit

When it comes to gluten cross-contamination in our food, it can take just a crumb (or for those who are particularly sensitive to trace gluten, even less) to induce nasty glutening symptoms.Many makeup and skin care products contain gluten ingredients (often in the form of hydrolyzed wheat protein, which is processed but not enough to remove all the gluten). So it only would take a taste of one of these products to potentially gluten you. Why take the risk?

What If I Want to Take the Risk?

Okay, so you love your products and you don't want to switch. I get it, I really do. Here's what you'll need to do (and not do) in order to stay safe while using gluten-containing makeup:

Do

Avoid gluten-containing lip products like the plague to avoid ingestion.

Wash your hands thoroughly, including under your nails (especially if you bite your nails), every time you touch a gluten-containing product.

Don't

Use a gluten-containing product anywhere near your mouth.

Use powders that contain gluten, since they could become airborne (inhaled gluten is a problem).

Rub your face and then touch your lips without washing your hands again first.

If you follow these rules, you should be able to eliminate as much risk as possible... and potentially pinpoint any symptoms you might have more quickly.

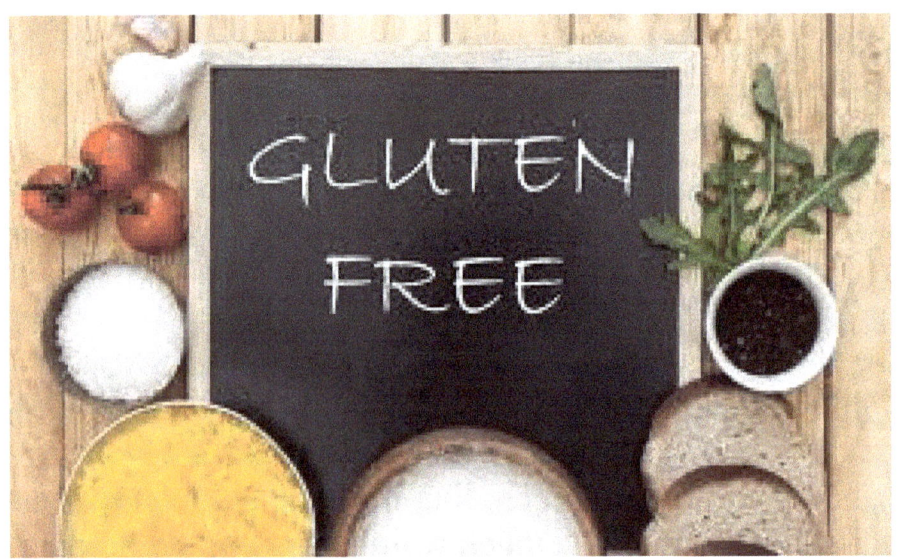

Gluten-Free Makeup Brands

To help you wade through the thicket of information and Latin ingredient names, we contacted a wide variety of makeup brands, both small and large, to ask about gluten ingredients in their products.

Below are makeup companies' statements on gluten (where provided), and our conclusions about whether you should feel confident using their products, should exercise caution, or should avoid them altogether. In most cases, the decisions will depend on how forthcoming the company has been about possible gluten ingredients, and how large a risk of gluten cross-contamination there is in the manufacturing of the products in question.

Here's our alphabetical list of makeup brands, plus what each brand has to say about the gluten content of its products.

Afterglow Cosmetics

Afterglow Cosmetics products are made in a gluten-free facility and are certified gluten-free by the Gluten-Free Certification Organization (GFCO), which requires products to meet stringent standards of less than 10 parts per million (ppm) of gluten (lower numbers are better). Afterglow Cosmetics uses Vitamin E (tocopherol) derived from organic cottonseed oil and organic olive oil (not from wheat germ, as is common in the cosmetics industry).

The bottom line: I would use anything from Afterglow Cosmetics without any hesitation—the products are completely safe for the gluten-free community.

Alima Pure

Alima Pure makes eco-friendly, mineral-based makeup that's cruelty-free. According to the company: "All of our loose powder products are gluten-free, as is our Lip Tint, Velvet Lipstick, and Natural Definition Mascara. However, only our loose powder products are created in a designated gluten-free facility."

The bottom line: You're perfectly safe to use any loose powder products from Alima Pure. Exercise caution with other products, especially if you're particularly sensitive to trace gluten.

Bare Minerals

This company states many of its products don't contain gluten, but it can't guarantee that they're gluten-free. They are made in a shared facility or on shared equipment. Many people with celiac disease and non-celiac gluten sensitivity do report using Bare Minerals products without issue.

The bottom line: Exercise caution, as Bare Minerals does not claim any products are gluten-free.

BITE Beauty

BITE Beauty, which makes only lip products, sells through Sephora. The company also offers BITE Beauty Lip Lab, a shop in SoHo in New York City that will custom blend lip products for you. The company's products are certified gluten-free.

The bottom line: BITE Beauty products are perfectly safe for those with celiac disease and gluten sensitivity.

CoverGirl

Here's the statement from Cover Girl: "If we add gluten, wheat or wheat extract directly to a product, it will be listed in the ingredients on the label. Still, we cannot give a 100% guarantee that trace levels of gluten are not present."

The bottom line: You'll have to check ingredients carefully on CoverGirl products to make sure gluten grain ingredients aren't present, and there's always the possibility of cross-contamination if you're particularly sensitive.

Ecco Bella

This is a safe brand for those of us with celiac or gluten sensitivity. From the company: "There is no gluten or wheat protein in any Ecco Bella product. All our products are safe for customers with celiac sprue."

The bottom line: I would try anything from Ecco Bella, and use it with confidence.

E.L.F.

This brand uses all gluten-free ingredients and also does not test on animals or use ingredients derived from animals, according to the company's statement. However, it does sometimes use shared equipment.

The bottom line: E.L.F. cosmetics are quite safe.

em michelle phan

This brand is made and marketed in partnership with L'Oreal. The company will not disclose whether or not gluten-based ingredients are used in its products.

The bottom line: You'll have to check ingredients carefully on em michelle phan products to make sure gluten grain ingredients aren't present, and there's always the possibility of cross-contamination. There are safer brands out there.

Gabriel Cosmetics

This all-natural, paraben-free line of cosmetics has been certified gluten-free by the GFCO, which requires products to include fewer than 10 parts per million of gluten. Gabriel Cosmetics also is vegan (with the exception of its makeup brushes, which are cruelty-free).

The bottom line: Anyone with celiac disease or gluten sensitivity can confidently order and use anything from Gabriel Cosmetics.

Lancome

This brand is owned by L'Oreal, so you should refer to the answer from L'Oreal, below.

Lili Lolo

Lili Lolo offers mineral makeup, including foundation, powder, blush, lip, and eye products. According to the company, everything in the Lili Lolo line is gluten-free except for the BB Cream, which contains wheat germ.

The bottom line: Definitely skip the BB Cream, but you should be able to use other products in the makeup line safely.

L'Oreal

This makeup conglomerate is not transparent when it comes to gluten-containing ingredients in its products.

The bottom line: If you really want to use a L'Oreal product, you'll have to check ingredients carefully to make sure gluten grain ingredients aren't present, and there's always the possibility of gluten cross-contamination even if you don't spot something that's obviously gluten-y. There are better choices available.

Maybelline New York

Maybelline also is owned by L'Oreal, so see the answer from L'Oreal directly above.

Mirabella Beauty

According to Mirabella, all its products except for its skin tint crème are gluten-free (there's wheat protein in the skin tint crème). Mirabella reports that its vendors test ingredients for trace gluten "and are AMAZINGLY thorough." Gluten-free products may be made in a shared facility, but Mirabella takes special care to clean the equipment in between batches. The company also doesn't perform animal testing.

The bottom line: Mirabella Beauty takes a careful approach to serving the gluten-free community. I wouldn't hesitate to try any product, with the exception of the gluten-containing skin tint crème.

NARS Cosmetics

A NARS customer service representative couldn't provide a list of gluten-free products.

The bottom line: I would steer clear of NARS Cosmetics products, since the company doesn't promise to disclose specific gluten-containing ingredients, and uses shared equipment.

Nivea

According to Nivea, gluten-containing ingredients in the company's products include: triticum vulgare (wheat bran), secale cereale (rye seed extract), hordeum vulgare (barley), and avena sativa (oat bran). Nivea adds that there's a risk of cross-contamination due to shared facilities.

The bottom line: You'll have to check ingredients carefully on Nivea products to make sure gluten grain ingredients aren't present. This isn't the best brand for anyone who's particularly sensitive.

NYX Cosmetics

This company does not provide ingredient information and does not pledge to disclose any gluten-containing ingredients.

The bottom line: I would steer clear of NYX Cosmetics products.

Pangea Organics

Pangea might not truly count as a makeup company—it makes three lip balms, but mainly creates beauty products such as cleansers, toners, and creams. However, the company is extremely careful when it comes to gluten. All of its products are considered gluten-free, with the exception of its Oatmeal Bergamot Bar Soap, which Pangea doesn't include on its gluten-free list because of the possibility of gluten cross-contamination in the oatmeal from nearby wheat fields. Pangea Organics also states that "our Vitamin E is sourced from either soy or sunflower, rather than wheat germ."

The bottom line: You can order anything from Pangea Organics with confidence (with the exception of the oatmeal soap).

Red Apple Lipstick

Despite the name, Red Apple Lipstick makes far more than just, well, lipstick. The company boasts lip pencils, lip balm, lip exfoliators, eye shadows, and eyeliners. All Red Apple products are gluten-free, with rigorous testing (aiming at zero parts per million of gluten) to ensure there's no trace gluten present. The company then follows that up with routine batch lab testing to ensure purity.

The bottom line: I would use anything from Red Apple Lipstick, including products designed for my lips, with confidence.

Revlon

Revlon does not test for gluten, nor does it provide any information on gluten-containing products.

The bottom line: I would steer clear of Revlon products.

Smashbox

This brand is a subsidiary of Estee Lauder. The company states that consumers can provide it with the name of individual products and that it will respond with information on those specific products. However, it will not provide consumers with an overall gluten-free list. Everything might be processed on shared equipment.

The bottom line: I would steer clear of any Smashbox products.

Too Faced Cosmetics

The company's entire line of cosmetics is gluten-free with the exception of our Borderline Lip Pencil, but products may be subject to cross-contamination in manufacturing. The company is cruelty-free and has an extensive vegan-friendly product list.

The bottom line: I'd feel comfortable using anything from Too Faced Cosmetics with the exception of the Borderline Lip Pencil.

Urban Decay

According to the company, some products do not include gluten ingredients, but Urban Decay does not test for trace gluten.

The bottom line: Urban Decay will tell you which products contain no gluten ingredients if you contact them at (800) 784-8722. We've used these products before, but always be aware of the possibility of gluten cross-contamination.

Zuzu Luxe

This brand, made by GFCO-certified Gabriel Cosmetics, also is certified gluten-free, which requires products to ensure they contain fewer than 10 parts per million of gluten. Most Zuzu Luxe products also are corn-free and vegan, according to the company.

The bottom line: Zuzu Luxe products are perfectly safe for people with celiac and gluten sensitivity to use.

Top 9 Gluten-Free Grains

There are more gluten-free grains than you probably would have guessed. Here are the top nine gluten-free grains I recommend, which also work as gluten-free flours. Most of these are fairly easy to find at your local grocer, and they're versatile and diverse enough to replace wheat in just about any recipe.

Amaranth: Amaranth offers digestive benefits and helps build healthy bones. It's a great source of protein, fiber, manganese, magnesium, phosphorus and iron.

Brown Rice: Can promote a healthy heart, provide manganese and decrease cholesterol.

Buckwheat: Buckwheat is a nutrient-dense seed filled with antioxidants.

Corn Grits (Polenta): Corn-based grains, like polenta, can be a great gluten-free source, but there is one key thing to consider: Is it non-GMO? Look for non-GMO versions and you will likely fare well due to the antioxidants and fiber they contain.

Millet: Millet is also a seed often referred to as a grain. Yes, birds love this little seed, and you, too, may want to give it a shot. Its fiber content and low glycemic index help keep the body regulated while maintaining healthy blood sugar levels.

Oats: Oats always seem to be in question as to whether they make the gluten-free list. So are oats gluten-free? The short version is, yes, oats are gluten-free, but they can be grown in the same fields as wheat products. That may be where a gluten sensitivity lies with oats, as the gluten remnants can find their way into oats. Purchase brands that label them as gluten-free. If needed, call the company to ask about how they're produced.

Quinoa: Quinoa has been very popular over the years due to its gluten-free status. Additionally, it contains protein, antioxidants, vitamins and minerals.

Sorghum: Sorghum is typically found as a flour and does well with nutrient density, offering protein, iron, B vitamins and dietary fiber. It also contains inflammation-reducing antioxidants.

Teff: You may not have heard of teff, but this gluten-free grain aids in circulation as well as weight loss.

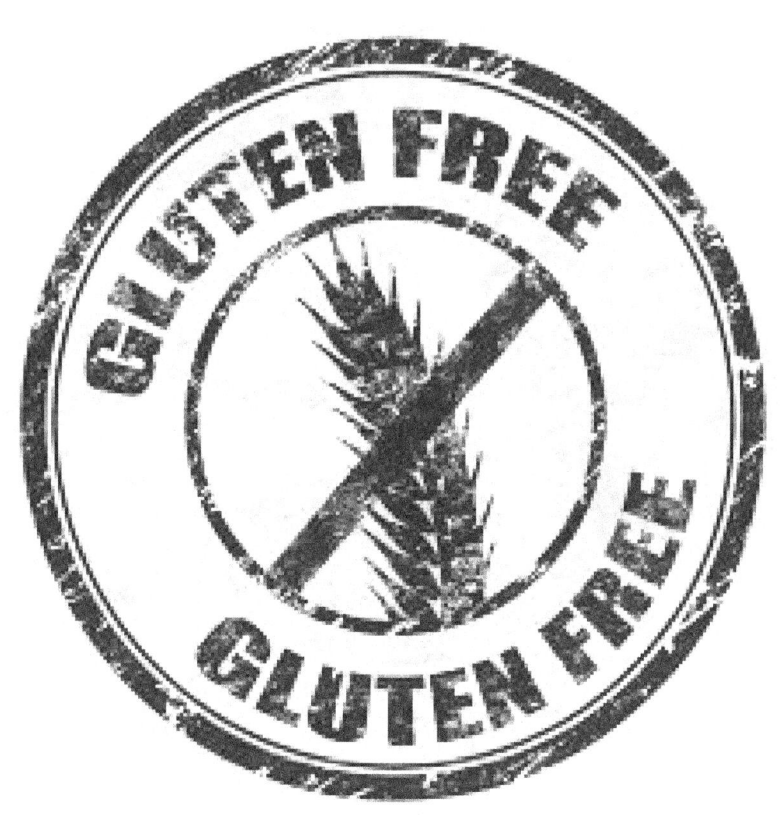

Top 3 Grains that Contain Gluten

Wheat is commonly found in:

- breads
- baked goods
- soups
- pasta
- cereals
- sauces
- salad dressings
- roux

Barley is commonly found in:

- malt (malted barley flour, malted milk and milkshakes, malt extract, malt syrup, malt flavoring, malt vinegar)
- food coloring
- soups
- beer
- brewer's yeast

Rye is commonly found in:

- rye bread, such as pumpernickel
- rye beer
- cereals

Gluten-Free Grains vs. Grains with Gluten

So with all this gluten-free buzz that has been around for quite a while, what does our body need? It's pretty clear that if you have celiac disease or a gluten intolerance, you have to steer clear of the sticky protein. However, for many gluten is simply a buzzword, and not having it could cause you to miss out on the benefits of many whole grains.

Some benefits include a lower risk of stroke, type 2 diabetes, heart disease, asthma, colorectal cancer, inflammatory diseases and gum disease, increased satiety, and healthier weight status. Whole grains, especially when produced properly and free of harsh chemicals, can offer vitamins and minerals, such as B6, E, niacin, pantothenic acid, riboflavin, thiamine, folate, calcium, iron, magnesium, zinc, copper, selenium and potassium, fiber, protein, antioxidants, health-protective phytonutrients and healthy fats. If you don't have problems digesting gluten, then you probably have no need to avoid it.

Regardless, the Chicago Tribune reports that there are ways to consume healthy gluten-free grains, but some gluten-free grains actually don't provide much nutritional value. Shelley Case, R.D., a dietitian, gluten-free diet expert and author of "Gluten-Free Diet: A Comprehensive Resource Guide," notes that many gluten-free foods are made from refined grains and starches, such as white rice flour, corn starch, potato starch or tapioca starch, that offer little in the nutrition department. Case — along with the USDA and the Whole Grains Council advises that those who regularly eat whole grains have lower disease rates.

So, if you're going to go gluten-free, opt for gluten-free grains that offer more nutrition than the ones mentioned by Case.

How to Include Gluten-Free Grains in Your Diet + Gluten-Free Grain Recipes

Looking for ways to incorporate gluten-free grains into your diet? Here are some ideas:

Make a blend of gluten-free grains, such as amaranth, buckwheat and brown rice, as a side dish or add to soups.

Add your favorite gluten-free grain, like quinoa, to soups or sprinkle over salads.

You can add amaranth or teff to brownies, cakes and cookies for added nutritional benefits and texture.

Cook extra gluten-free grains to make a hearty breakfast cereal. Just add some banana or fresh fruit, a drizzle of honey, a few nuts, and a sprinkle of cinnamon.

You can blend them into a great vegan or vegetarian burger with black beans, gluten-free rolled oats, or cooked brown rice, quinoa, amaranth or teff.

Gluten-free grains recipes

Paleo Tortillas Recipe Corn-Free with Healthy Oils
INGREDIENTS:

- 2 eggs
- 1 cup full-fat, canned coconut milk
- 1 tablespoon avocado oil
- ¾ cup arrowroot starch
- 3 tablespoons coconut flour
- ¼ teaspoon salt

DIRECTIONS:

Preheat the oven to 300 F.

In a mixing bowl, combine the wet ingredients and mix until well-combined.

Add the dry ingredients to the bowl and mix well.

Drizzle avocado oil in a small skillet over medium to medium-low heat.

Pour ⅓ cup of batter into the pan, using a spatula to spread it out.

Allow tortilla to cook for 2–3 minutes then flip, cooking for another 2–3 minutes.

Keep them warmed in the oven until all tortillas are made and ready to use.

When you walk through the grocery store, I'm sure you notice the array of tortillas available. There's flour tortillas, whole wheat tortillas, corn tortillas and more. Most of these products are made with processed, refined ingredients that are stripped of the nutrients we seek when preparing a healthy meal.

My Paleo tortillas are different. They are completely free of gluten and GMO corn; plus, they contain healthy alternatives like coconut milk and arrowroot starch. You'll never settle for buying store-bought tortillas again when you see how easy it is to do it yourself. Plus, you know exactly what's going into your food — no hidden or genetically modified ingredients here! Try these Paleo tortillas with any of these taco recipes or my healthy chicken fajitas. I know you won't be disappointed!

Slow Cooker Chicken and Rice Recipe
INGREDIENTS:

- 2 chicken breasts, diced
- 1 white onion, diced
- 2 cups sprouted brown rice
- ½ tablespoon salt
- ½ tablespoon pepper
- 1 tablespoon garlic
- ½–1 cup shredded goat cheese
- 4½–5 cups chicken bone broth

DIRECTIONS:

Add everything to the slow cooker and cook on low for 8 hours.

One of the most-used tools in my kitchen is the slow cooker. It's the great cooking equalizer even if you have no experience cooking, slow cooker chicken recipes allow you to just dump all the ingredients, let the pot do its magic and have a delicious meal ready several hours later. One of my favorite go-to recipes is this slow cooker chicken and rice.

Crockpot chicken and rice ingredients
A Healthier Chicken and Rice

Chicken and rice is super simple to make. This slow cooker recipe is pretty basic, so it's great for picky eaters, but it's also super flavorful and healthy. I always make chicken and rice with brown rice. White rice is a refined carbohydrate, which has no nutritional value. These types of carbs enter the bloodstream like sugar, triggering the release of insulin. What happens next is that your body converts the sugar into stored fat rather than energy.

Crockpot chicken and rice step 1

Brown rice is a complex carbohydrate, so it resists immediate breakdown. Instead, the body breaks it down and converts the food into sugar over time. The two don't taste significantly different, either, but brown rice is 1,000 times better for you.

Along with the chicken and rice, you'll use chicken bone broth instead of plain old water. The bone broth is one of the best things you can consume for leaky gut, digestion issues and boosting the immune system, and it works perfectly in this crockpot chicken and rice.

How to Make Slow Cooker Chicken and Rice

If you're ready to make this fool-proof chicken and rice, let's get started.

Crockpot chicken and rice step 2

Start by dicing both the onions and chicken.

Crockpot chicken and rice step 3

I used boneless, skinless chicken breast here, but you could easily swap in boneless, skinless chicken thighs instead.

Crockpot chicken and rice step 4

Next, add all of the ingredients to the slow cooker.

Crockpot chicken and rice step 5

Yes, that includes the cheese! This goat milk cheese will add a little extra flavor to this dish.

Crockpot chicken and rice step 6

Finally, step away from the slow cooker. Go to the gym, get some work done, go shopping. When you return to the crockpot in 8 hours, dinner will be ready and waiting!

Spinach Mushroom Quiche
Ingredients

- Crust
- 1 cup Bisquick™ Gluten Free mix
- 1/3 cup plus 1 tablespoon shortening
- 3 to 4 tablespoons cold water Filling
- 1 tablespoon butter
- 1 small onion, chopped (1/3 cup)
- 1 1/2 cups sliced fresh mushrooms (about 4 oz)
- 4 eggs
- 1 cup milk
- 1/8 teaspoon ground red pepper (cayenne)
- 3/4 cup coarsely chopped fresh spinach
- 1/4 cup chopped red bell pepper
- 1 cup gluten-free shredded Italian cheese blend (4 oz)

Steps

1 Heat oven to 425°F. In medium bowl, place Bisquick mix. Cut in shortening, using pastry blender (or pulling 2 table knives through ingredients in opposite directions), until particles are size of small peas. Sprinkle with cold water, 1 tablespoon at a time, tossing with fork until all flour is moistened and pastry almost leaves side of bowl (1 to 2 teaspoons more water can be added if necessary).

2 Press pastry in bottom and up side of ungreased 9-inch quiche dish or glass pie plate. Bake 12 to 14 minutes or until crust just begins to brown and is set. Reduce oven temperature to 325°F.

3 Meanwhile, in 10-inch skillet, melt butter over medium heat. Cook onion and mushrooms in butter about 5 minutes, stirring occasionally, until tender. In medium bowl, beat eggs, milk and red pepper until well blended. Stir in spinach, bell pepper, mushroom mixture and cheese. Pour into partially baked crust.

4 Bake 40 to 45 minutes or until knife inserted in center comes out clean. Let stand 10 minutes before cutting.

Expert Tips

A 4-oz can of sliced mushrooms (drained) can be substituted for the fresh mushrooms. If you prefer, you can use gluten-free shredded Cheddar or gluten-free shredded Monterey Jack cheese in place of the Italian cheese blend.

Gluten-Free Impossibly Easy Breakfast Bake

Ingredients

- 1 package (16 oz) bulk gluten-free pork sausage
- 1 medium red bell pepper, chopped
- 1 medium onion, chopped
- 3 cups frozen hash brown potatoes
- 2 cups shredded Cheddar cheese (8 oz)
- 3/4 cup Bisquick™ Gluten Free pancake & baking mix
- 2 cups milk
- 1/4 teaspoon pepper
- 6 eggs

Steps

1 Heat oven to 400°F. Spray 13x9-inch (3-quart) glass baking dish with cooking spray. In 10-inch skillet, cook sausage, bell pepper and onion over medium heat, stirring occasionally, until sausage is no longer pink; drain. Mix sausage mixture, potatoes and 1 1/2 cups of the cheese in baking dish.

2 In medium bowl, stir Bisquick™ mix, milk, pepper and eggs until blended. Pour over sausage mixture in baking dish.

3 Bake 30 to 35 minutes or until knife inserted in center comes out clean. Sprinkle with remaining 1/2 cup cheese. Bake about 3 minutes longer or until cheese is melted. Let stand 5 minutes before serving.

Expert Tips

Cooking Gluten Free? Always read labels to make sure each recipe ingredient is gluten free. Products and ingredient sources can change.

Peanut Butter Banana Pancakes

Wake up to warm peanut butter banana pancakes, a sweet twist on the traditional pancake. Filled with chopped bananas and peanut butter, these pancakes couldn't be easier to make! Just add Bisquick™ Gluten-Free mix, water, sugar, salt and an egg – and your peanut butter ...

Ingredients

- 1 1/4 cups Bisquick™ Gluten Free mix
- 1 1/2 cups warm water
- 1/2 cup creamy gluten-free peanut butter
- 1/4 cup granulated sugar
- 1/8 teaspoon salt
- 1 egg
- 1/2 cup chopped banana (about 1 small)
- 1 sliced banana, if desired
- 1/4 cup powdered sugar, if desired

Steps

1 Heat griddle or skillet over medium heat (375°F). Brush with vegetable oil if necessary or spray with cooking spray without flour before heating. In medium bowl, stir Bisquick mix, warm water, peanut butter, granulated sugar, salt and egg with whisk. Fold in chopped banana.

2 For each pancake, pour 1/4 cup batter onto hot griddle. Cook 2 to 3 minutes or until bubbles form on top and edges are dry. Turn; cook other side until golden brown. Top pancakes with sliced banana; sprinkle with powdered sugar.

Expert Tips

Pancakes are ready to turn when they are puffed and bubbles form on top

Mix pancake batter in a measuring cup or bowl with handle and spout. Then you can easily pour batter onto griddle

For tender pancakes, mix just until dry ingredients are moistened. There may still be lumps in the batter.

Keep pancakes warm in a single layer on paper towel-lined cookie sheet in a 200°F oven.

Always read labels to make sure each recipe ingredient is gluten free. Products and ingredient sources can change.

Zucchini-Ribbon "Lasagna"

Ingredients

For the Sauce (makes 3 cups)

- 1 can (28 ounces) whole peeled plum tomatoes, with juice
- 2 tablespoons extra-virgin olive oil
- 1 small onion, finely chopped (1 cup)
- 1/4 teaspoon red-pepper flakes
- 12 ounces ground turkey, preferably dark meat

- 2 tablespoons chopped fresh oregano
- 2 teaspoons coarse salt

For the Lasagna

- 2 medium zucchini, trimmed
- 1 cup part-skim ricotta cheese
- 1/4 teaspoon extra-virgin olive oil
- Freshly ground pepper
- Garnish: Fresh oregano

Directions

Step 1

Make the sauce:

Pulse tomatoes with juice in a food processor until finely chopped. Heat oil in a large straight-sided skillet over medium heat. Cook onion and red-pepper flakes, stirring occasionally, until onion is tender, about 8 minutes. Add turkey; cook, breaking up any large pieces, until browned, 3 to 4 minutes. Add tomatoes; bring to a boil. Reduce heat; simmer until thick, about 20 minutes. Stir in oregano and salt. Let cool.

Step 2

Make the lasagna:

Preheat oven to 375 degrees. Slice zucchini lengthwise into thin strips (about 1/8 inch thick) using a mandoline or a sharp knife. Place 5 or 6 zucchini slices, overlapping slightly, in the bottom of an 8-inch square baking dish. Top with 1 cup sauce. Dot with 1/4 cup ricotta. Repeat twice with zucchini, remaining sauce, and 1/2 cup ricotta, alternating direction of zucchini. Top with remaining zucchini, alternating direction; brush with oil. Dot with remaining 1/4 cup ricotta. Season with pepper. Bake,

uncovered, until lasagna bubbles and top browns, 50 to 60 minutes. Let stand for 10 minutes. Garnish with oregano.

Cauliflower Pizza Crust

Ingredients

1/2 head cauliflower, coarsely chopped1/2 cup shredded Italian cheese blend1/4 cup chopped fresh parsley1 egg1 teaspoon chopped garlicsalt and ground black pepper to tasteAdd all ingredients to list

Directions

Place cauliflower pieces through the feeding tube of the food processor using the grating blade; pulse until all the cauliflower is shredded.

Place a steamer insert into a saucepan and fill with water to just below the bottom of the steamer. Bring water to a boil. Add cauliflower, cover, and steam until tender, about 15 minutes. Transfer cauliflower to a large bowl and refrigerate, stirring occasionally, until cooled, about 15 minutes.

Preheat an oven to 450 degrees F (230 degrees C). Line a baking sheet with parchment paper or a silicon mat.

Stir Italian cheese blend, parsley, egg, garlic, salt, and pepper into cauliflower until evenly incorporated. Pour mixture onto the prepared baking sheet; press and shape into a pizza crust.

Bake in the preheated oven until lightly browned, about 15 minutes.

Nutrition Facts

Per Serving: 59 calories; 3.5 g fat; 3.3 g carbohydrates; 4.3 g protein; 38 mg cholesterol; 109 mg sodium. Full nutrition

CPSIA information can be obtained
at www.ICGtesting.com
Printed in the USA
BVHW062318110521
607047BV00012B/2650